RESISTANT STARCH MANUAL

The Complete Guide to Resistant Starch

HYDIE THIESFIELD

Table of Contents

CHAPTER ONE

A Starch That's Resistant

The Complete Guide to Resistant Starch

There are a lot of starches in your diet.

Long chains of glucose found in grains, potatoes, and many other foods are known as "starches."

It's important to note, however, that not all of the starch you consume is absorbed.

In some cases, you may not even notice that it has passed through your digestive system.

In other words, it is unable to be absorbed by the human body.

Resistant starch is a type of starch that works like soluble fiber.

Resistant starch has been shown to have powerful health benefits in numerous human studies.

Improved insulin sensitivity, decreased blood sugar, decreased appetite, and various digestive advantages are all part of this.

These days, resistant starch is a hot topic. In the past, many people have experimented with it and found significant results by incorporating it into their daily diets.

Starch Resistant to Heat and Light

There are many varieties of resistant starches. In total, there are four varieties.

Grains, seeds and legumes contain Type 1, which is difficult to digest because of the cell walls' fibrous structure.

There are two types of starchy foods that contain Type 2: raw potatoes and unripe green bananas.

Cooking and cooling starchy foods, such as potatoes and rice, results in Type 3. Through retrogradation, some of the digestible starches are transformed into resistant starches (3).

Resistant starch is not so simple to categorize because it can exist in the same food in a variety of forms.

The amount of resistant starch in a food depends on how it is prepared.

Reducing the resistant starches in a banana by letting it ripen (turn yellow) will result in regular starches.

To What End?

Resistance starch works because it acts like soluble, fermentable fiber. "

Undigested, it reaches your colon, where it nourishes your friendly gut bacteria and aids digestion.

Despite the fact that your body's cells outnumber the gut flora by ten to one, you're only 10% human.

Fermentable fibers and resistant starches, on the other hand, feed 90% of your cells while most foods only feed 10%.

Bacteria in your intestines come in a wide variety of forms. A growing body of evidence suggests that the number and type of bacteria in your body has a significant impact on your health.

The beneficial bacteria in your intestine are fed by resistant starch, which increases both the diversity and abundance of the bacteria there.

In the process of digesting resistant starches, bacteria produce gases and short-chain fatty acids, most notably butyrate.

A Nutritional Powerhouse for Your Body's Gut.

Reducing the amount of short-chain fatty acids in your bloodstream is an important part of a healthy diet.

In terms of importance, butyrate is the most important of these short-chain fatty acids.

The cells that line your colon prefer to run on butyrate as a fuel source instead of glucose.

Resistant starch, on the other hand, feeds both friendly bacteria and the cells in your colon by boosting butyrate levels.

CHAPTER TWO

Colon health is aided by resistant starch in a number of ways.

Colorectal cancer is the fourth most common cause of cancer death in the world, and reducing the pH level, reducing inflammation, and resulting in a number of beneficial changes should reduce your risk.

It's possible that the short-chain fatty acids that aren't used by colon cells travel through your bloodstream to your liver and other parts of your body, where they can have various beneficial effects.

Resistant starch may help treat a variety of digestive disorders because of its therapeutic effects on the colon. Some examples of these include ulcerative colitis, Crohn's disease, diverticulitis and diarrhea.

Resistance starch has also been found to enhance mineral absorption in animal studies.

There is still a lot of work to be done before any strong recommendations can be made about butyrate's role in health and disease.

Resistant Starch's Health Benefits

The metabolic health benefits of resistant starch are numerous.

Insulin sensitivity, or the ability of cells in your body to respond to insulin, has been shown in several studies to be improved by this method.

After a meal, resistant starch can help lower blood sugar levels by acting as a blood sugar stabilizer.

To top it all off, resistant starch has a second meal effect, meaning that eating it for breakfast lowers your blood sugar spike for lunch as well.

It has a significant impact on glucose and insulin metabolism. Insulin sensitivity can be improved by up to 50% after just four weeks of consuming 15–30 grams of carbohydrates per day.

There aren't enough words to describe how important it is to have high levels of insulin sensitivity.

Many serious diseases, including metabolic syndrome, type 2 diabetes, obesity, heart disease, and Alzheimer's, are thought to be linked to low insulin sensitivity (insulin resistance).

Resistant starch may help you live longer and stay healthy by increasing insulin sensitivity and lowering blood sugar levels.

Resistant starch, on the other hand, may not be as beneficial as previously thought. The dose and type of resistant starch all play a role.

The ability to feel fuller for longer periods of time may help with weight loss.

In terms of calories per gram, resistant starch is less calorie-dense than regular starch.

Having more resistant starch content in a food means that it has a lower caloric content.

Soluble fiber supplements have been shown in a number of studies to aid in weight loss by increasing satiety and decreasing appetite.

The same effect can be seen with resistant starch. People eat fewer calories when resistant starch is included in their meals.

It's been found that resistant starch can help animals lose weight, but this hasn't been proven in human studies.

Tips for Eating More Resistant Starches

Resistant starches can be added to your diet in two ways: either by eating them, or by taking a supplement.

Resistant starch is found in a number of everyday foods.

There are a variety of raw and cooked potato options, as well as green and yellow bananas, various beans and nuts, and raw oatmeal.

Since all of these foods are high in carbohydrates, they aren't an option if you're following a very low carbohydrate diet.

But if you are on a low-carb diet with carbs in the 50–150 gram range, you can eat some of it

It is possible, however, to include resistant starch in your diet without increasing the amount of digestible carbohydrates you consume. Many people have suggested supplements like raw potato starch for this purpose.

Approximately 8 grams of resistant starch are found in

each tablespoon of raw potato starch.

Furthermore, it is extremely affordable.

It has a mild flavor and can be consumed in a variety of ways, including sprinkled on food, dissolved in liquid, or blended into drinks.

Resistant starch can be found in four tablespoons of raw potato starch, which should yield 32 grams. To avoid flatulence and discomfort, it's best to begin slowly and gradually increase your dosage.

As long as you don't exceed the recommended daily intake of between 50 and 60 grams, you won't have any problems.

Short-chain fatty acids can take up to four weeks to build up in your body and reap the benefits, so be patient.

CHAPTER THREE

Resistant Starch Calories

Although resistant starch contains calories, the amount is significantly lower than that found in regular starch.

When resistant starch makes it to the colon, the bacteria there turn it into fuel. Short-chain fatty acids are the end product of a process known as fermentation (SCFAs). These fatty acids are responsible for the vast majority of the calories and numerous health benefits that resistant starch provides.

Soluble fiber and oligosaccharides also produce SCFAs. On some food labels, the amount of calories associated with some fiber is listed. These calories, on the other hand, do not raise blood sugar.

Advantages for Your Health

Researchers are discovering more and more health benefits associated with resistant starches as their research expands. Resistant starch and oligosaccharides and fermentable fiber both share many of the same health benefits.

Butyrate

Butyrate, a type of SCFA, is particularly associated with resistant starch. Butyrate has been found to be protective of colon cells and associated with a lower risk of cancer, according to research.

Cells also benefit from butyrate in a variety of ways. Resistant starch has a major advantage over oligosaccharides and soluble fiber in this regard.

Butyrate is produced by their fermentation, but not to the same extent as resistant starch.

Absorption of minerals.

Resistant starch, like other fermentable fiber, is linked to improved mineral absorption. Resistant starch consumption has been shown in animal studies to improve intestinal absorption of calcium and magnesium. 1 Be aware that these studies were conducted on animals and further research is needed to determine the effects on humans.

Insulin sensitivity has been improved.

Resistant starch appears to improve insulin sensitivity, which is particularly exciting for people with diabetes.

Fermentable fiber and resistant starch have been linked to improved glucose tolerance in the "second meal effect," which can occur the following meal or the following day.

2

A peptide produced during the fermentation process may be to blame for this, according to the evidence.

Satiety

The release of a different peptide may be a factor in the increased satiety caused by resistant starch (PYY). After eating, your appetite is suppressed for about 12 hours by the hormone Peptide YY, which is produced in the intestines.

Resistant starch has been studied in both normal weight and obese subjects. Publicly available research shows that it has the ability to increase satiety and reduce both hunger and food intake. 3

Additional Advantages

Resistant starch's positive effects on health are being studied by scientists. There are numerous health benefits associated with its consumption, including lower cholesterol and triglyceride levels, improved bowel regularity, and an increase in "good" bacteria in the gut.

Resistance starch in food may be linked to less fat storage post-meal, researchers are looking into this.

Resistant Starch-Positive Foods

Resistant starch can be found in a wide variety of foods, which you can include in your diet.

Beans and legumes are both examples of legumes.

The amount of resistant starch in different types of beans (and preparation methods) varies. A good rule of thumb is that most beans contain about an equal amount of slow-digesting and resistant starch.

Resistant starch can be obtained from these sources:

• Peas

• Lentils

Beans in White

However, products like Beano, which improves the digestibility of beans, will also reduce the amount of resistant starch in the food.

Potatoes, Rice, and Other Grains

Resistant starch can be found in a variety of starchy foods, including whole grains and potatoes.

• Bulgar Wheat

cooked and cooled oatmeal

Overcooked and cooled down potatoes are included here.

white or brown rice that has been cooled down after being cooked

• Barley, pearl

• Oats that have not been cooked (such as in overnight oats)

Bananas that are green in color.

For the most part, the majority of us prefer to consume bananas that have been allowed to ripen to their fullest potential. Bananas lose their resistant starch as they ripen, which is a pity. Resistant starch is also lost if you cook bananas.

Instead, buy green bananas and eat them within two to three days if you can.

Resistant starch is abundant in plantains.

Starch made from potatoes

To increase their intake of resistant starch, some people take potato starch as a supplement. Only if the white flour-like powder is not cooked can it be used in smoothies or other dishes.

A Variety of Other Delicacies

Resistant starch is another benefit of maize corn starch. It can be used in baked goods as a substitute for some of the flour. It results in a softer, more airy feel.

The Bottom Line

To break a weight loss plateau, lower blood sugar, improve digestion, or simply experiment with yourself, resistant starch might be a good option for you to consider.

THE END

www.ingramcontent.com/pod-product-compliance
Lightning Source LLC
Chambersburg PA
CBHW050817160726
48004CB00002B/885